Mosby's

Psychiatric Nursing Study Guide

Mosby's

Psychiatric Nursing Study Guide

Lynette W. Jack, PhD, RN, CARN
Assistant Professor
School of Nursing
University of Pittsburgh
Pittsburgh, Pennsylvania

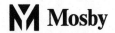 Mosby

St. Louis Baltimore Boston Carlsbad Chicago Naples New York Philadelphia Portland
London Madrid Mexico City Singapore Sydney Tokyo Toronto Wiesbaden

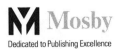

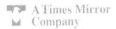

Dedicated to Publishing Excellence

A Times Mirror
Company

Publisher: Nancy L. Coon
Editor: Jeff Burnham
Developmental Editor: Linda Caldwell
Project Manager: Gayle Morris
Production Editor: Gina Keckritz
Design and Layout: Ken Wendling
Designer: Dave Zielinski
Manufacturing Manager: Dave Graybill

Copyright © 1997 by Mosby-Year Book, Inc.

Printed in the United States of America
Composition by Wordbench

Mosby-Year Book, Inc.
11830 Westline Industrial Drive
St. Louis, Missouri 63146

International Standard Book Number: 0-8151-5285-X
28747

97 98 99 00 01/9 8 7 6 5 4 3 2 1

Preface

Psychiatric Nursing is an exciting and challenging specialty. You will have an opportunity during this course to learn much about yourself and to develop interpersonal skills that will help you with all your interactions with people. You will understand human behavior more fully. Within this course, you will learn about various mental disorders and the appropriate nursing interventions to help people manage these illnesses.

This study guide will help you to be an active learner. The benefit of active learning is that you understand the content more fully and remember it longer than when you are a passive learner who simply sits in class and listens to a lecture. Use of the worksheets in this study guide will give you an opportunity to apply psychiatric nursing concepts to clinical situations and case studies; as a result, your knowledge and skills will be greatly enhanced.

To use this study guide effectively, you will need to read the chapters in your textbook associated with each content area and listen to the instruction you receive in the classroom before you complete the worksheets. Your instructor may assign specific worksheets as homework or may use some of the worksheets as the basis for discussion or small-group work within the classroom. Some of the worksheets can be used individually, whereas others are best used as discussion guides so that you can hear the ideas, opinions, and strategies of your classmates to enrich your own learning.

Many different learning activities are contained in these worksheets, including:

case studies
scrambled word exercises
matching exercises
fill-in-the-blank questions
short answer questions
crossword puzzles
label-the-diagram exercises
nursing care plans
critical thinking questions
discussion questions
community assessments
personal assessments
client record reviews

Much of what we know about psychiatric illnesses and nursing's response to them has changed in the past 10 to 15 years, especially as we have learned more about the biological dimensions of these illnesses. However, many aspects of psychiatric nursing—and what we know is therapeutic within a nurse-client relationship—have remained classic and central features of this specialty. The worksheets in this study guide will help you to learn about the newest information as well as the classic concepts.

Enjoy your learning in this course. You will find this information applicable no matter where you practice nursing, and the skills you begin to develop during this course will be an asset to you and your clients as well.

Lynette W. Jack

Table of Contents

Chapter 1 Introduction to Psychiatric Nursing

ACTIVITY 1   Name _____

List the standards of psychiatric-mental health clinical nursing practice published by the American Nurses Association and give an example of a behavior a nurse would display that matches each standard. You do not need to include the standards reserved for specialist practice.

Standard I:

Standard II:

Standard III:

Standard IV:

Standard V:

Standard Va:

Standard Vb:

Standard Vc:

Standard Vd:

Standard Ve:

Standard Vf:

Standard Vg:

Standard Vk:

Chapter 1 Introduction to Psychiatric Nursing

ACTIVITY 2   Name _____

Discussion Questions: Within your class or your clinical group, discuss your answers to these questions. As an alternative to group discussion, if that opportunity is not available to you, you may write your answers to the questions directly on this worksheet.

1. Describe mental health and compare its characteristics with those of mental illness or mental disorder.

2. How has the delivery of psychiatric-mental health nursing changed? Comment on changes in roles, functions or activities, and settings.

3. What issues or trends must be of concern to psychiatric nurses who plan to practice beyond the year 2000?

Critical Thinking Exercise

Construct a health care system which meets the mental health and psychiatric needs of the people within the region it serves. Describe the following:

  a. characteristics of the region you choose and the people in it;
  b. services available in your health care system;
  c. roles and services you see psychiatric nurses providing; and
  d. strategies you will use to ensure access to needed services, quality of care, and cost effectiveness.

Chapter 2 Theoretical Models

ACTIVITY 1   Name _____

Indicate "T" for True and "F" for False.

_____ 1. Rational emotive therapy focuses primarily on the expression of feelings.

_____ 2. A person's perception or appraisal of a stressful situation determines his or her response to the stress.

_____ 3. When a psychiatrist talks about the client's conflict between id impulses and superego values, she is using the psychoanalytic model.

_____ 4. If a person does not master the basic tasks during adevelopmental stage, he can never function effectively or learn those skills at a later time.

_____ 5. According to Hildegard Peplau, a major role for the psychiatric nurse is reality orientation to enable the client to learn to adjust his thought patterns to meet reality.

_____ 6. Peplau used Erikson's stages of development as a critical part of her framework in the interpersonal theory of nursing.

_____ 7. Cognitive techniques assist clients to notice their own automatic negative thoughts and the connection of those thoughts to moods and actions.

_____ 8. Thought stopping and progressive relaxation are behavioral techniques useful in managing reactions to anxiety-provoking situations.

_____ 9. *Coping* refers to a person's efforts to master demands that are perceived as exceeding the person's resources.

_____10. Interpretation of dreams and transference phenomena are techniques used by a therapist using a psychoanalytic model.

Chapter 2 Theoretical Models

ACTIVITY 2   Name _____

1. Match the DSM-IV axis with its description:

   _____ Axis I   a. medical diagnoses

   _____ Axis II   b. global assessment of functioning

   _____ Axis III   c. psychosocial, environmental stressors

   _____ Axis IV   d. major psychiatric disorder

   _____ Axis V   e. personality disorder

2. Match the following pieces of data about a client with the appropriate axis from DSM-IV:

   _____ Axis I   a. being treated for Parkinson's Disease

   _____ Axis II   b. has been unable to locate an apartment with easy
                                       access for someone with limited mobility

   _____ Axis III
                                   c. has daily panic attacks

   _____ Axis IV
                                   d. symptoms severely interfere with daily
   _____ Axis V   functioning

                                   e. has been avoiding people for most of his life
                                       because of fear of criticism

3. Review charts in the clinical setting and record here the DSM-IV information for one of the
   clients. Then, briefly summarize the client's reason for admission or treatment.

   Axis I:

   Axis II:

   Axis III:

   Axis IV:

   Axis V:

   Summary of client's presenting problem:

Chapter 2 Theoretical Models

ACTIVITY 3

Name _____

....

Match the example in Column A to the name of the defense mechanism in Column B.

Column A

1. _____ A woman who is attracted to her doctor communicates with him in a sarcastic, hostile manner.
2. _____ Mary's employer tells her she has a drinking problem that is interfering with her job performance; later she tells her family that her boss said her work was good.
3. _____ A woman who has beaten her mother then develops excessive hand-washing behavior.
4. _____ Susan talks about being assaulted with no apparent emotion.
5. _____ John says he failed the test because his teacher wrote bad test questions.
6. _____ Allison failed to make the cheerleading squad, then worked hard academically, becoming an honor student.
7. _____ Greg fails a test and "forgets" to tell his parents.
8. _____ Meg was severely criticized by her head nurse; when she got home, she started a fight with her husband.
9. _____ Sam experienced a lot of stress at work, so he went to bed, curled up in a tight ball, and slept for a couple of days, missing work.
10. _____ A woman who spent too much money shopping goes into an extensive explanation of the benefits of her purchases and how much money she saved by buying what she did.
11. _____ Mike says he was drinking while underage because his friends made him do it.
12. _____ Mrs. Brown was in a severe automobile accident and cannot remember any details about what happened.
13. _____ A young man who was in trouble a lot as an adolescent goes on to become a police officer.
14. _____ Through several self-awareness exercises, Karla realizes that she is modeling herself after a well-respected instructor.
15. _____ A little boy scolds his toys while playing, and his mother realizes that he sounds just like her.

Column B

a. compensation

b. denial

c. displacement

d. dissociation

e. identification

f. intellectualization

g. introjection

h. projection

i. rationalization

j. reaction formation

k. regression

l. repression

m. sublimation

n. suppression

o. undoing

Chapter 2 Theoretical Models

ACTIVITY 4   Name _____

Critical Thinking Questions

You have been assigned to work with a 19-year-old college student who has requested help because she has been experiencing multiple minor physical complaints, including headaches, stomach aches, backaches, occasional chest pain and tachychardia, and fatigue. The treatment team has determined that this client's symptoms are related to stress.

1. Use a stress/adaptation model to explain what is happening to this client.

2. What strategies or nursing interventions would be appropriate in working with this client if you were using the stress/adaptation model?

3. How would your approaches to the client's problems change if you were using an interpersonal model?

4. Using the concepts of mental health and therapeutic use of self, describe your own strengths and limitations in working with this particular client.

Chapter 3 Therapeutic Communication

ACTIVITY 1   Name _____

Matching: Draw a line from the communication technique in Column B to the nurse response from Column A matching that technique.

Column A

"Don't worry. Everything will be OK."

"I know how hurt you must have felt."

"So your mother remarried soon after you were born."

"You seem uncomfortable when you talk about your family."

"Why do you feel this way?"

"No one here would lie to you. This hospital has a fine reputation."

"Maybe this is something you and I can figure out together."

"I'm not sure I follow. Can you tell me more about that?"

"Why don't you try talking more openly with your husband?"

"I hear what you are saying. Go on."

"It sounds as if you might be bored at home."

"Everyone has problems at times. You just have to keep going."

Column B

seeking clarification

minimizing problems

empathizing

defending

verbalizing the implied

offering false reassurance

general lead

placing event in time or sequence

making observations

advising

suggesting collaboration

requesting an explanation

Now, circle the therapeutic communication techniques.

Name _____

Circle the letter of the one answer you think is the most therapeutic response to the client statement.

1. "I feel so sad. I don't think I can go on anymore."
   a. "Don't worry about it so much. Things will look better in the morning."
   b. "Perhaps a warm bath would help."
   c. "Things must seem very difficult for you right now."
   d. "You're not thinking of killing yourself, are you?"

2. "I don't feel like talking to you anymore."
   a. "All right then. Go to lunch."
   b. "You're not working very hard today. We might as well stop."
   c. "Are you angry with me about something?"
   d. "You don't want to talk any more right now?"

3. "Give me your phone number, and we'll get together when I leave the hospital."
   a. "My instructor doesn't allow me to give out my number."
   b. "I don't date patients."
   c. "You've got to be kidding!"
   d. "I appreciate your trust in me, but ours is a nurse-client relationship."

4. "This has been a dismal day."
   a. "Yes, I know. I feel the same way."
   b. "Go on."
   c. "Don't be silly! See how bright the sun is shining."
   d. "Cheer up! Things will get better!"

5. "I've been in the hospital for two days, and no one has paid any attention to me."
   a. "That's not true. I've been here three times already."
   b. "Well, the nurses are very busy today."
   c. "Everyone's ignored you?"
   d. "What do you mean?"

6. "The doctor comes in and out so fast that he doesn't take time to listen to me."
   a. "He does the best he can. He's a busy man."
   b. "What did you want to tell him?"
   c. "He tells you what you need to know."
   d. "That's for sure. He doesn't even answer our questions!"

7. "You know, the food is really rotten here."
   a. "You don't like the food?"
   b. "What's the matter with it?"
   c. "Would you like to try cooking for this many people?"
   d. "Yes. I sure wouldn't want to eat it."

8. "I feel like I'm going to cry."
   a. "You look sad."
   b. "Please don't cry."
   c. "Now, now."
   d. "Everything is going to be all right."

9. "Get away from me. You're all trying to hurt me."
   a. "You're in the hospital. We're only trying to help you."
   b. "You must be feeling frightened."
   c. "Settle down or I'll have to call security."
   d. "You'll feel better after your family visits."

10. "Just leave me alone, and let me die."
    a. "Don't be silly. I can't do that."
    b. "Of course. We're all going to die."
    c. "What do you mean, you're going to die?"
    d. "You seem upset. Tell me what's bothering you."

Name _____

Critical Thinking Questions

1. Your client asks you to explain why he gets so angry when he tries to talk to his family. You hear his voice getting louder and his speech is rapid and pressured. You begin to feel unsure of yourself and a little frightened. Describe the factors that may be influencing your communication with this client, and tell how you will respond to him.

2. Under what circumstances is self-disclosure therapeutic, and under what circumstances would it be inappropriate?

3. What does confrontation mean? Give some guidelines for making clinical decisions about whether to use confrontation when working with a client.

Chapter 3 Therapeutic Communication

ACTIVITY 4   Name _____

This activity is based on the video "Basic Principles for Communicating Effectively" from Mosby's Communication in Nursing Video Series.

1. Verbal communication involves two parts: vocabulary skills and speaking skills.
   a. True
   b. False

2. Give four examples of therapeutic techniques.

3. Give three examples of nontherapeutic techniques.

4. Which therapeutic technique assists the client in separating the relevant parts of the conversation from the irrelevant?
   a. planning
   b. restating
   c. silence
   d. summarizing

5. Silence provides an opportunity for the client and the nurse to collect their thoughts.
   a. True
   b. False

6. What cannot be avoided when sending a verbal message?
   a. giving advice or opinions
   b. being defensive or judgmental
   c. sending nonverbal messages
   d. none of the above

7. When used in a reassuring, gentle way in a therapeutic environment, which of the following will show the client that you care?
   a. parallel communication
   b. nonverbal communication
   c. touch
   d. none of the above

8. Which of the following factors influence how clients interact?
   a. environment
   b. purpose of communication
   c. nurse-client relationship
   d. individual's past experience
   e. all of the above

9. Which therapeutic technique will provide the nurse with more information and go beyond a yes-or-no response?
   a. knowing the purpose of the interaction
   b. controlling distracting environmental factors
   c. maintaining good eye contact and periods of silence
   d. none of the above

10. When the nurse is able to concentrate on what the client is saying, is positioned to face the client, and feels comfortable in continuing his or her thoughts, the nurse is engaging in:
    a send nonverbal messages.
    b. preparing verbal messages.
    c. therapeutic communication.
    d. active listening.
    e. a, c, and d

Chapter 4 Nurse-Client Relationship

ACTIVITY 1   Name _____

....

Write in the blank the term that best describes the component of a nurse-client relationship illustrated by each scenario. Use the following list of terms.

self-awareness	genuineness
rapport	therapeutic use of self
warmth	respect
empathy	concreteness
immediacy	confrontation

Scenario #1   _____

Mr. Johnson is working with a nurse therapist to learn how to manage his feelings without the use of alcohol. His alcohol dependence has been a priority in his life, at the expense of his relationships with his family. He has described to the nurse many situations that show how he has hurt his wife and daughters. The nurse therapist conveys unconditional acceptance of Mr. Johnson as a person, while working with him to help him heal old emotional wounds in his family.

Scenario #2   _____

The nurse demonstrates to the client that she is able to put herself in the client's place in order to understand the situation from the client's point of view.

Scenario #3   _____

The nurse shares an experience from his past to illustrate that he honestly understands what the client is trying to say. He tells the client that he is sincerely interested in working with her to find a solution to the client's problem.

Scenario #4   _____

The client, Susan, is describing her depression and has been using vague, general statements about being sad all the time. The nurse says, "Can you tell me specifically how your sad feelings interfere with your daily activities?"

Scenario #5   _____

Amy's psychiatric nursing instructor has given an assignment in which Amy is to examine her own personality, thoughts, feelings, and perceptions. The purpose of this assignment is to help Amy increase one area of her interpersonal skills.

Chapter 4 Nurse-Client Relationship

ACTIVITY 2   Name _____

Match each activity in Column A to the stage in the nurse-client relationship when the activity is most appropriate.

Column A   **Column B**

1. _____ Explore personal beliefs and feelings.   a. preorientation/design

                                                            b. orientation/warm-up

2. _____ Review feelings about the relationship.   c. agreement/contracting

3. _____ Discuss how often meetings will occur.   d. working/rehabilitation

                                                            e. termination/finishing

4. _____ Determine what the client needs.

5. _____ Formulate a working pact.

6. _____ Overcome resistance behaviors.

7. _____ Mutually set goals.

8. _____ Evaluate progress toward goals.

9. _____ Review appropriate theory.

10. _____ Gather comprehensive data about client.

11. _____ Help client learn new behaviors.

12. _____ Bring an end to the relationship.

13. _____ Finalize referral for further treatment.

14. _____ Help client become comfortable talking about concerns.

15. _____ Plan for first interaction with client.

Chapter 4 Nurse-Client Relationship

ACTIVITY 3   Name _____

Discussion Questions: Within your clinical group or in the classroom, discuss the following questions. If this approach is not possible, write out your own individual answers directly on this worksheet.

1. What are the differences between a friendship or social relationship and a therapeutic nurse-client relationship?

2. What should you do when you find yourself reacting in a very strongly emotional way to a client you have been interacting with? What might be responsible for your feelings? Give an example of a client who might arouse strong feelings in you.

3. You have been working with a client for two weeks, and you feel good about the level of trust that has been established between the two of you. Today the client tells you that he is suicidal, and he demands that you promise not to tell anyone else or he will stop trusting you. What will you do?

ACTIVITY 4   Name _____

....

Critical Thinking Exercise

Kathy and Mary are two teen-aged clients who have been attending the intensive outpatient day treatment program where you are assigned for your clinical learning experiences in psychiatric/mental health nursing. You have enjoyed interacting comfortably with both of them and find them to be a lot like your younger sister's friends. They have been talking about pranks they pulled on teachers in school, fights they have had in their neighborhood, and times they have stolen merchandise from the local stores. They have confided to you that they regularly smoke marijuana and cigarettes, and you have shared some stories about your high school days.

Today, when Kathy and Mary enter the day treatment center, they seem especially happy. Their speech is loud and somewhat slurred, and they go from person to person around the room, laughing and poking the others, getting too close to some people. You can see that some clients are getting upset, and one older client has threatened to hit Kathy. You go over to the two girls, hoping to intervene and convince them to get involved in some constructive activity. When you approach, both girls push you aside and run out of the center, laughing and using profanity all the way out the door. You smell the odor of alcohol as they push you aside.

Explain the dynamics of this nurse-client relationship. How do you react to the two clients now, compared with how you initially felt about them? What changes might be made in the relationship to deal with today's events? What have you learned about nurse-client relationships? Use additional paper to answer this if necessary.

Name _____

Place each piece of data listed below under its correct category found on one of the following three pages for a comprehensive assessment.

Data:

asking if she has chronic fatigue syndrome
slowed movements
crying at times during interview
no evidence of hallucinations or delusions
expressing feelings of helplessness
has been feeling sad almost every day for past month
unable to get up in morning and get to work on time
chronic headaches
chest pain
normal EKG
being treated for psoriasis
aware of time, place, person
works as an insurance claims adjuster
few words, slowed responses to questions
says she can't go on like this anymore
was treated for depression twice before
does not currently take any medication
neat and clean, well-groomed
normally a good housekeeper, but hasn't been interested or "up to it" lately
argues with husband a lot about how much he works
son died of accidental overdose 6 months ago
college degree in accounting
stopped going to church when son died
cooperative with questioning during interview
has lost 20 pounds in last 2 months
sleeps no more than 3-4 hours per night
used to take Tofranil
smokes 1 pack per day and drinks 1-2 glasses wine each evening
says she doesn't know what's happening to her
talks in monotone, soft voice
mother was treated for depression
talks logically, with no display of emotion

current medical problems	mood/affect

general appearance and behavior	previous psychiatric history

mental status exam	current medications

family history	perceptions

cognitive functioning	insight

culture	coping skills/mechanisms

spirituality	psychosocial/environmental factors

problems	relationships

thought content/processes	speech

ACTIVITY 2   Name _____

....

Read each case study and formulate nursing diagnoses based on the data in the case study.

Case #1

    Mrs. Jackson is 32 years old, married, and has two children, ages 3 and 5. She is requesting help because she says she feels nervous all the time. She sometimes avoids going to the grocery store because she worries that something really terrible will happen and she will be trapped inside. Mrs. Jackson has been having a hard time sleeping at night because of her worries, and is tired all day, which makes caring for her two children very difficult. She says she really hates herself because she feels incompetent and stupid all the time.

Nursing diagnoses:

  1.

  2.

  3.

Case #2

    JoAnn has been separated from her husband for 6 months, and she no longer sees her parents either. She says they all complained that she was drinking excessively and should stop, but she couldn't stop because she needed to drink every day in order to handle all the stresses of her job. She has been worried lately because a lot of people are being laid off, and she thinks she may not be as qualified for her job as some of the other people she works with. She says she has been shy and self-conscious all her life and thinks that her problems began when she was verbally and physically abused by her alcoholic father. Now she says she feels frightened, disconnected from everyone and everything, and overwhelmed by hopelessness.

Nursing Diagnoses:

  1.

  2.

  3.

Chapter 5 Nursing Process

ACTIVITY 3   Name _____

Read each nursing diagnosis and identify expected outcomes.

1. Anxiety related to inability to manage feelings of anger, as evidenced by frequent headaches and stomach aches, verbal outbursts at family members, social isolation, and generalized worries without an identifiable cause.

      short-term goal(s):

      long-term goal(s):

2. Altered thought processes related to discontinuation of phenothiazines as evidenced by hallucinations.

      short-term goal(s):

      long-term goal(s):

3. Hopelessness related to severity of physical problems and lack of curative medical care, as evidenced by pronounced sadness, verbalized feelings of helplessness and hopelessness, lack of comfort from spiritual resources, and inability to participate actively in group therapy.

      short-term goal(s):

      long-term goal(s):

Read the following case study and develop a nursing care plan, using the blank forms on the next pages. Two forms have been provided for different nursing diagnoses.

Mrs. D is a 51-year-old African-American woman who presents with concern about depression and anxiety. She tells the nurse that she has been having difficulty sleeping and has felt sad for the past three months. Currently, she is caring for her husband, who has inoperable stomach cancer, and her 13-year-old grandson, who has attention deficit hyperactivity disorder. She worries that something will happen to her and that she will be unable to care for them. She says they need her and will never get along without her. She is preparing for the time when her husband dies, and she is feeling very sad. Her current symptoms include difficulty getting to sleep and staying asleep, daytime fatigue, social withdrawal, psychomotor retardation, excessive guilt, tearfulness, decreased concentration, and feelings of worthlessness. She denies suicidal ideation but does indicate that she wouldn't mind just not waking up some mornings. She keeps going because of her responsibilities to others.

Mrs. D has been treated for depression and anxiety before and has taken several antidepressants and some antianxiety medication. She can't remember the names of the medications. She first was treated for severe nightmares, in which big black monsters were coming to kill her. She says she knows that these relate to traumatic events in her childhood that she has not resolved. Her difficulties have been so severe that she has been unable to work. In the past, she had been a successful attorney and health care lobbyist.

Mrs. D currently takes Klonopin, prescribed by her family doctor to help with her anxiety. She has been treated frequently for angina and also at one time had a seizure disorder. She has been seizure-free for the past three years.

One of the greatest concerns that Mrs. D has is that she has few coping skills for dealing with the stressors in her family. She also worries that she has not resolved old issues from childhood and currently has difficulty completing activities of daily living because of her symptoms of depression. She is willing to take medication if it will help, but she believes that she would most benefit from a therapy relationship.

Nursing Care Plan

Nursing Assessment Data

Nursing Diagnosis

Outcomes

    Short-term goals

    Long-term goals

Interventions   **Rationale**

Nursing Care Plan

Nursing Assessment Data

Nursing Diagnosis

Outcomes

    Short-term goals

    Long-term goals

Interventions   **Rationale**

Chapter 6 Psychobiology

ACTIVITY 1   Name _____

Label the major structures of the brain in this figure and indicate the functions associated with each area.

Include the following structures:

corpus callosum	limbic system
frontal lobe	hypothalamus
temporal lobe	medulla
reticular formation	cerebellum
thalamus	occipital lobe
parietal lobe	sensory strip
motor strip.	

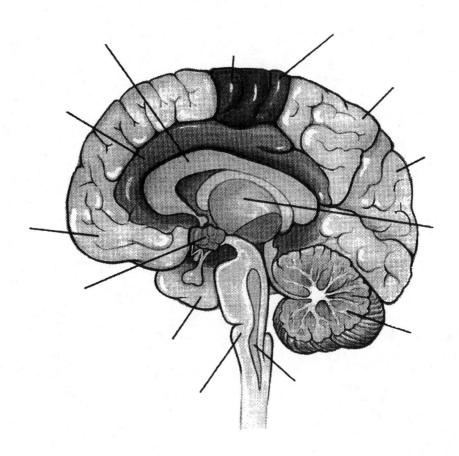

ACTIVITY 2   Name _____

Define or explain each term.

1. cerebellum

2. synapse

3. peripheral nervous system

4. hypothalamus

5. basal ganglia

6. magnetic resonance imaging (MRI)

7. computerized tomography (CT)

8. electroencephalography (EEG)

9. positron emission tomography (PET)

10. cerebral blood flow (CBF)

Chapter 6 Psychobiology

ACTIVITY 3   Name _____

....

Short Answer

1. What mental illness has been associated with excesses of the neurotransmitter dopamine? Explain.

2. Explain the changes in neurotransmitters associated with mood disorders.

3. How is panic disorder related to changes in brain chemistry?

4. Explain the biological changes associated with Alzheimer's disease.

ACTIVITY 4   Name _____

....

Critical Thinking Exercise

Mrs. Anderson is a 48-year-old woman who is being treated for bipolar disorder via her fifth hospitalization in the past 15 years. She has experienced both depressive and manic phases of the illness. Her daughter, Susan, has asked you to explain what is happening to her mother. Susan is 19 years old and is in a serious relationship with a college classmate. She wonders aloud whether she, too, will have problems with her mood and whether she should consider marriage and having children. What will you say to her?

Chapter 7 Sociocultural Aspects of Psychiatric Nursing

Critical Thinking Exercise

1. Develop questions that a nurse should ask of herself or himself to complete a self-assessment of cultural competence.

2. Talk to members of your family about your own cultural heritage. Write a description here of what you learn about your own culture, your values, communication patterns, health beliefs, time and space orientation, religion, and any other information that helps to define you as a person from a particular culture.

3. Compare your discoveries about your own cultural background with the information a classmate has learned about himself or herself.

Critical Thinking Exercise

Formulate at least 15 questions you would ask when doing a cultural assessment of a client.

....

Critical Thinking Exercise: Read the case study and answer the questions that follow.

You work as a staff nurse on an acute psychiatry unit in a large hospital in Chicago. Your assignment includes providing care for Mary, a 36-year-old African-American who has been sent to the unit with a diagnosis of schizophrenia, paranoid type. Her chart reveals that she lights candles and places them under her bed to scare away evil spirits. She is apparently on leave from her job, where she said she put a curse on a co-worker who had angered her. Mary is highly agitated, with restless pacing. She was given Haldol in the emergency room, just before they brought her up to the unit. Mary was accompanied to the hospital by her sister, who explained that the family grew up in Jamaica and moved to Chicago when Mary was in high school. The sister warns that they are a close family and that more than 10 of them will come to visit Mary while she is in the hospital. On the unit, Mary has been screaming that she sees the devil coming after her. She also displays symptoms of tardive dyskinesia but says that this is a part of the "spell the devil done" and refuses to let you give her any additional medication. She is hard to understand because she speaks in a dialect that is not familiar to you.

1. What problems can you identify in this case about Mary?

2. What assumptions do you make about Mary, based on what you know about her sociocultural background?

3. What further information do you need to obtain via a cultural assessment?

4. What medication issues have occurred that may be related to Mary's cultural heritage?

5. How will you adapt your nursing care plan to reflect your sensitivity to Mary's culture?

Critical Thinking Exercise

You work in a large urban hospital that treats clients predominantly from a poor inner city neighborhood, with many ethnic minorities represented in the population. How can you develop mental health services that are culturally sensitive for the clients you serve? Describe the sociocultural issues that have an impact on the development of such services. What kinds of programs would you propose to develop to meet the mental health needs of your clients?

Chapter 8 Legal and Ethical Issues

Name _____

Describe each of the following types of entry into psychiatric/mental health treatment:

1. voluntary admission

2. involuntary admission

3. emergency admission

4. outpatient commitment

When the law says that a client has the right to treatment in the *least restrictive environment*, what does that mean?

1. List client rights as they are protected by law.

2. Record in the blank provided the client right that is being violated in each situation.

   a. _____

   Two nurses are talking about a patient in the elevator, calling the patient by both first and last names. The elevator is crowded with people, including families.

   b. _____

   The unit is short-staffed today. One of the patients is a wanderer, so the staff ties him in a chair so that they don't have to watch him every minute.

   c. _____

   A patient has been screaming, and the staff is getting annoyed with this behavior, so the nurse draws up an injection to calm the patient. The patient says he doesn't want the medicine beause it makes him too drowsy, but the nurse says it's for his own good, and she gives it anyway.

   d. _____

   A patient has been on a long-term unit at the state mental hospital for years, where she works well in the patient laundry. She is not required to attend any groups and does not see a counselor, but instead goes to work every day.

Name _____

Short Answer

1. How can a nurse determine what information must be documented in a client's record?

2. What is the benefit of detailed documentation?

3. List five specific things that should be documented in a client's record.

4. How does proper grammar, spelling, and use of abbreviations play a role in effective charting?

Chapter 8 Legal and Ethical Issues

ACTIVITY 4   Name _____

....

Critical Thinking Exercise

A man is brought to the emergency room after the police picked him up while he was wandering through the streets of a high-crime neighborhood muttering unintelligibly. He has long, shaggy hair and an unkempt beard, and there is no identifying information on him. He refuses to tell anyone what his name is, and he swings his fists at people who come close to him. Although most of his speech is incoherent, it is possible to hear the words "kill" and "gun" periodically. Most of the ER staff are frightened that he will do something to hurt himself or someone else in the ER. The decision is made to give this man an injection of Haldol to help calm him. When the nurse comes toward him with the syringe, he starts screaming "No, no!!"

1. What should the nurse do in this situation?

2. What are the man's legal rights?

3. What alternatives to giving the injection might there be?

The man is admitted to the psychiatric unit on an emergency commitment. He is medicated and bathed, and within several days he is beginning to behave appropriately, although he still appears to be responding to voices. When the emergency commitment expires, the treatment team realizes that there is insufficient evidence of danger to self or others to hold this man in the hospital. They try to link him into an outpatient aftercare program but are told that he will have to come in for an intake assessment. He is given an appointment in two weeks. The man is discharged and given information about a homeless shelter nearby, along with an appointment card for his outpatient assessment. A week later, the police who originally brought him into the hospital drop by to tell you that he has been found dead. He apparently shot himself with a gun.

4. What ethical dilemmas are raised by this situation?

5. How does the organization of the mental health care system play a role in what happened to this man?

6. How do you feel about what has been described in this case study?

Chapter 9 Psychiatric Nursing in the Community

ACTIVITY 1   Name _____

Discussion Questions: Within your clinical group or in the classroom, discuss the following questions. If this approach is not possible, write your own individual answers to these questions about psychiatric treatment in the community.

1. Describe deinstitutionalization and its impact on communities and clients with severe and persistent mental illness.

2. What services were mandated by the Community Mental Health Act of 1963?

3. For each of these levels of prevention, describe mental health services that may be provided within the community.

    a. primary prevention

    b. secondary prevention

    c. tertiary prevention

4. Describe the role(s) of the psychiatric nurse working in the community.

ACTIVITY 2   Name _____

Choose a community that you are familiar with. List examples of the following resources within the community and assess their availability, accessability, affordability, and cultural appropriateness.

1. General community resources (education, clean environment, safety, streets, recreation, etc.)

2. Community health resources (health care providers, emergency services, support groups, wellness programs, etc.)

3. Community mental health resources (community mental health centers, support programs, housing, vocational rehabilitation services, agencies for vulnerable populations, etc.)

Case Study: Read the following case description and answer the questions below.

Jan is a home health nurse scheduled to make her first home visit to a client with a diagnosis of chronic obstructive pulmonary disease. The client is Mrs. Annabelle Adams, who is a 63-year-old widow, living in the 3-story home where she and her late husband raised their six children. Mrs. Adams has never worked and has been a widow for the past three years, since her husband died very suddenly of an acute myocardial infarction. She currently requires oxygen, which she gets from a portable tank and a nasal cannula. She is 5' 3" tall, weighs 265 pounds, and admits to smoking 2 packs of cigarettes per day. She says the food and cigarettes help her to stay calm, since three of her children are living with her, along with 3 young grandchildren, whom Mrs. Adams babysits while their mother goes to work. Mrs. Adams says that sometimes she gets so worried about everything that she feels sharp chest pain, along with severe headaches and dizziness. When asked what she worries about, she says that one of her boys keeps getting into trouble when he drinks too much and one of her daughters has been in the hospital recently after taking too many pills.

1. List the problems you can identify from the data provided.

2. What additional data would you collect?

3. Describe three interventions that you would implement.

4. What community resources might be helpful to Mrs. Adams and her family?

Critical Thinking Exercise

Describe the knowledge and skills needed by a psychiatric nurse case manager working in a community mental health center in a densely populated neighborhood of a large metropolitan area.

How can this psychiatric nurse case manager work to provide a seamless continuity of care?

1. Unscramble the trade name of the psychotropic medication using the clue provided.

a. E T R I Z H A N O

_____

an antipsychotic medication helpful in managing acute agitation

b. X I P A L

_____

an antidepressant useful in managing depression in the elderly because of its few cardio-
vascular side effects

c. T A P A E N R

_____

antidepressant requiring careful monitoring of
diet during administration

d. O T N G C E N I

_____

medication added to treat drug-induced
extrapyramidal symptoms

e. R I P L I O N X E A A D O T C N E

_____

available in long-acting injectable form for
control of symptoms associated with schizophrenia

f. T I L U H M I

_____

most commonly prescribed medication for
mania

2. Draw a line from the generic name in Column A to that medication's trade name in Column B.

Column A	Column B
benztropine	Benadryl
fluphenazine	Mellaril
risperidone	Cogentin
haloperidol	Risperdal
thioridazine	Haldol
diphenhydramine	Prolixin
clozapine	Thorazine
phenelzine	Prozac
paroxetine	Depakene
fluoxetine	Desyrel
imipramine	Clozaril
lorazepam	Pamelor
valproic acid	Paxil
chlorpromazine	Nardil
nortriptiline	BuSpar
alprazolam	Ativan
trazedone	Tofranil
chlordiazepoxide	Librium
buspirone	Xanax

3. Match the medication in Column A with its corresponding classification from Column B.

Column A

_____ Clozaril

_____ Prozac

_____ Akineton

_____ Luvox

_____ Lithane

_____ Klonopin

_____ Zoloft

_____ Marplan

_____ Valium

_____ Tegretol

_____ Serzone

_____ Artane

_____ Sinequan

_____ Serax

_____ Depakote

_____ Risperdal

_____ Ambien

_____ Loxitane

_____ Effexor

_____ Navane

Column B

a. Antipsychotic

b. Antidepressant

c. Antianxiety agent

d. Mood stabilizer

e. Antiparkinson/antidyskinetic agent

Chapter 10 Psychopharmacology and Other Biological Therapies

ACTIVITY 2   Name _____

....

Using a term from the list below, label each scenario with the psychotropic medication side effect being described.

hypertensive crisis   neuroleptic malignant syndrome
acute dystonia   tardive dyskinesia
pseudo-parkinsonism   orthostatic hypotension
akathisia   agranulocytosis

Scenario #1 _____

Mr. Taylor was started on a high potency antipsychotic medication last evening because of severe and frightening hallucinations. He is late in getting up for breakfast this morning, and when he does get up, he complains of dizziness, darkness around the edges of his peripheral vision, and a "rush of warmth" to his head.

Scenario #2 _____

Nancy was given her first dose of Haldol 30 minutes ago. You hear a scream and leave the nurses' station to find Nancy at your doorway, wide-eyed and appearing very frightened. Her head is stiffly turned so that her chin is resting on her left shoulder, and she is calling out for help because she cannot turn her head.

Scenario #3 _____

Members of the stabilization group are complaining about Tom's jitteriness in group sessions. They say he is constantly moving, and they are beginning to feel anxious while near him. You ask Tom to describe what he is experiencing, and he tells you he isn't sure, but he knows that since he started taking that new medication, he hasn't been able to sit still.

Scenario #4 _____

Gary has been taking Haldol for one week. Today when you make morning rounds, you find that Gary is rigid, with hand tremors. He seems somewhat confused and his temperature is 103°. He is also displaying frequent, shallow respirations.

Scenario #5 _____

Joe Harris is a 72-year-old man with a long history of treatment for schizophrenia. He attends the day treatment center, and can regularly be observed making unusual facial grimaces, tongue movements, and lip smacking.

Chapter 10 Psychopharmacology and Other Biological Therapies

ACTIVITY 3   Name _____

1. List five key teaching points you would include when your client begins taking Clozaril.

   a.

   b.

   c.

   d.

   e.

2. List five key teaching points you would include when your client starts taking a monoamine oxidase inhibitor (MAOI) for treatment of depression.

   a.

   b.

   c.

   d.

   e.

3. List five key teaching points you would include when your client starts taking lithium.

   a.

   b.

   c.

   d.

   e.

4. List five key teaching points you would make when your client starts taking nortriptiline.

   a.

   b.

   c.

d.

e.

5. List five key teaching points you would make when your client starts taking an antianxiety medication.

a.

b.

c.

d.

e.

6. List five key points you would include in preparing your client for ECT.

a.

b.

c.

d.

e.

Critical Thinking Questions

1. What are the psychiatric nurse's responsibilities prior to starting a client on a psychotropic medication?

2. Noncompliance with medication regimens is a major contributor to relapse. Discuss factors which increase the likelihood of noncompliance and describe interventions which are likely to increase the client's compliance.

3. Identify ethical issues which must be addressed when ECT is being considered as a treatment strategy for a client.

Chapter 11 Working with the Family

ACTIVITY 1   Name _____

Read the following characteristics of families and label as either "F" for functional or "D" for dysfunctional.

_____ 1. feeling of need for each other and for others beyond the family

_____ 2. members' need for each other present only in a crisis

_____ 3. conflict expressed openly and frequently

_____ 4. weak and ineffective parental coalition

_____ 5. regular exercise and recreation

_____ 6. feelings attended to

_____ 7. mistrust of people beyond family

_____ 8. anger expressed through hitting and abuse

_____ 9. conflict over family rules and norms

_____ 10. final decisions made by parents

_____ 11. hopeful, positive outlook

_____ 12. coercion, punishment used by parents to get children to do right thing

_____ 13. power diffuse and centered in children

_____ 14. autonomy discouraged

_____ 15. strong element of control in caring

_____ 16. hopelessness predominant

_____ 17. communication unclear (incongruency between verbal and nonverbal)

_____ 18. little empathy shown

_____ 19. encouragement to express different ideas

_____ 20. links to society through work, play, school, church

_____ 21. prepared for loss and able to handle it

_____ 22. absence of dangerous activities

_____ 23. rigid or disordered quality

_____ 24. no significant health problems

Chapter 11 Working with the Family

ACTIVITY 2   Name _____

1. List difficulties that families face when there is a member with a mental illness.

2. Describe the impact of mental illness on the family.

3. Describe interventions that are helpful for families dealing with mental illness in a family member.

4. Name one resource for families dealing with mental illness that exists in your area, and describe the services that the resource provides.

Chapter 11 Working with the Family

ACTIVITY 3   Name _____

Critical Thinking Exercise

You are working as a staff nurse on a psychiatric unit in a small, community-oriented general hospital. You have been asked to develop a series of classes that would be helpful to families in the community, related to aspects of mental illness, the needs of those with mental illness, and the needs of families who have a member with mental illness. Describe the content of 10 sessions you would include in this series of classes.

Critical Thinking Exercise

Develop at least 15 questions you could ask to help you in assessing a family that has requested family therapy because of acting-out behaviors and school problems in their 9-year-old and 13-year-old children.

Chapter 12 Working with Groups

ACTIVITY 1   Name _____

1. List some benefits to clients that can be realized as a result of participation in a group.

Match the description of therapeutic factors associated with group participation as defined by Yalom with the name of that factor.

2. _____ altruism

3. _____ catharsis

4. _____ instillation of hope

5. _____ imparting of information

6. _____ imitative behavior

7. _____ interpersonal learning

8. _____ universality

a. The group provides varied opportunities for relating to other people and testing new ways of relating in a safe environment.

b. New knowledge is shared with members on such topics as medications, interpersonal skills.

c. There is an outpouring of emotional tension through verbalization of display of feelings during session.

d. The opportunity to support and share information and skills with another reduces preoccupation with self and increases self-esteem.

e. Progress in others is observed, and members of group feel optimistic that they, too, will improve.

f. Group member realizes that others share similar feelings or have similar problems.

g. group leader is a valuable role model for learning interpersonal skills.

Chapter 12 Working with Groups

Name _____

Explain the purpose and the focus of each of the following types of groups, and indicate what kinds of clients the group might help.

1. task groups

2. self-help groups

3. teaching/education groups

4. supportive therapy groups

5. psychotherapy groups

6. peer support groups

Chapter 12 Working with Groups

ACTIVITY 3   Name _____

Discussion Questions: Within your clinical group or in the classroom, discuss your answers to the following questions. If this approach is not possible, write your own individual answers directly on this worksheet.

1. What factors related to the inpatient setting influence group leadership techniques and responsibilities?

2. Describe the group leader's responsibilities for providing a physical setting that is conducive to an effective group meeting.

3. When would co-leadership of a group be a good idea? What problems might be anticipated when groups have co-leaders? How can co-leaders work effectively together?

4. Describe group rules or norms that the leader should state from the beginning and reinforce as the group continues to meet.

5. List three effective techniques a group leader could use to help the group become cohesive.

ACTIVITY 4   Name _____

....

Critical Thinking Exercise

You have been asked to start an inpatient group for the following patients:

  Tom, 32: diagnosed with schizophrenia, undifferentiated type; admitted 2 days ago

  Sam, 67: diagnosed with major depression, recurrent; admitted with psychomotor agitation 3
      days ago

  Mary, 40: diagnosed with schizophrenia, disorganized type; admitted two days ago with symp-
      toms of flat affect and disorganized speech

  Susan, 37: diagnosed with dysthymia; admitted 2 days ago with some suicide ideation but no
      plan

  Jennie, 29: diagnosed with major depression, single episode; admitted 3 days ago with sleep
      disturbance, anhedonia, anergia, lack of appetite, and profound hopelessness

  Mike, 62: retired steelworker who has been depressed since retirement on disability following
      an accident that caused head trauma

  Richard, 35: diagnosed with schizophrenia, paranoid type; readmitted today because of non-
      compliance with medication routine

1. List several types of groups that would be appropriate for these patients.

2. Choose one of the groups you have identified, then write goals for the group as a whole and
   for each of the patients in the group.

3. What problems might you anticipate in the group process?

4. How can you structure the group so that it is most likely to be effective?

5. How will you evaluate the group's effectiveness?

Chapter 13 Crisis Intervention

ACTIVITY 1   Name _____

Label each scenario with the type of crisis being described: *situational* or *maturational*.

1. _____

   Susan and John have just given birth to their first baby, who was born 8 weeks prematurely. The baby is in the NICU.

2. _____

   Jason is 10 months old and has just begun walking. His parents have not yet realized how much this will change the safety of his environment.

3. _____

   Marilyn has begun experiencing symptoms of menopause and is displaying some symptoms of depression as well, because she had been thinking about having another baby.

4. _____

   Sam has been abused, both emotionally and physically, by his father for the past 6 months, ever since his father lost his job. Sam is having difficulty in school and has started getting into fights.

5. _____

   Alexandra is 11 years old and has just started menstruating. She is uncomfortable about the changes in her body and has been avoiding all her friends from school.

6. _____

   Bob is seeking counseling because he is feeling stressed. He is 19 years old and has recently finished technical school and taken a job in an automobile repair shop. He feels as though he can't please his boss and has also started to fight with his girlfriend of two years.

7. _____

   Marion is a 72-year-old woman who has been experiencing more frequent health problems during the past two years. Her eyesight is failing, and she has cardiac and urinary problems that make it almost impossible to go out and enjoy herself.

8. _____

   Bob has been displaying symptoms of depression, and his Employee Assistance Counselor at work has sent him to a mental health center for an evaluation. Bob admits that he has been depressed since his wife filed for divorce several months ago.

9. _____

Christina has had symptoms of schizophrenia for more than ten years. She has been in and out of mental hospitals several times and resists taking medication on a consistent basis. Recently, she withdrew into her bedroom and refused to eat because she believed that the food her parents were bringing her was poisoned.

10. _____

Allison is a 16-year-old who has been sent to the counseling center by the school nurse, who noticed that Allison seemed to be unusually thin. With careful assessment, it is determined that Allison is displaying behaviors associated with an eating disorder, and she herself says that she has to be thin so that she will get invited to the prom.

Name _____

Fill in the boxes that help to explain Aguilera's model of crisis and balancing factors.

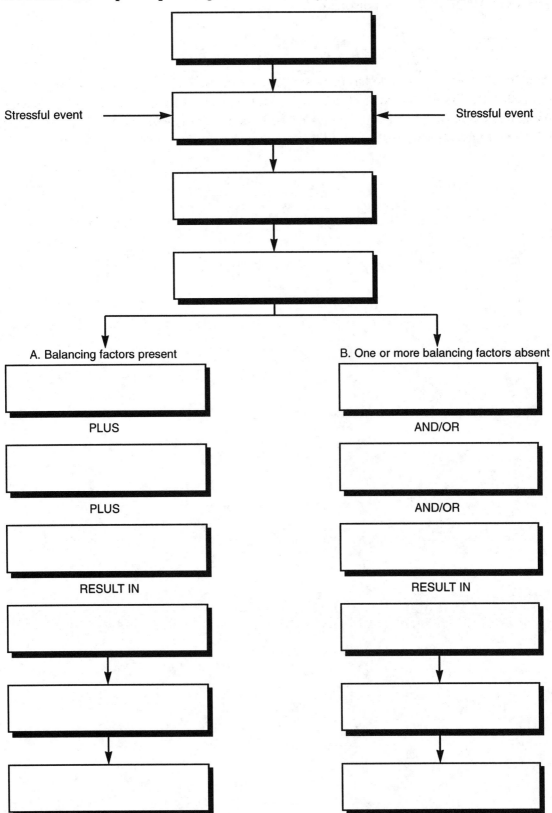

Stressful event →

Stressful event ←

A. Balancing factors present

PLUS

PLUS

RESULT IN

B. One or more balancing factors absent

AND/OR

AND/OR

RESULT IN

Name _____

Describe the steps in crisis intervention, explaining what occurs with each step.

1.

2.

3.

    a.

    b.

    c.

    d.

4.

Chapter 13 Crisis Intervention

ACTIVITY 4   Name _____

....

Critical Thinking Exercise: Read the following case study and describe how you would help the client deal with the crisis.

Tom is a 38-year-old factory worker who has been sent to the emergency room because of an injury to his right forearm, which occurred at work. His arm has been badly mangled, and it will have to be cleaned and a cast applied. However, Tom is screaming and seems highly agitated, not letting anyone near him. He is threatening to hurt anyone who tries to touch his arm. You are a member of the hospital's Crisis Intervention Team, and you are called to the ER to help Tom and the staff there resolve this problem so that necessary treatment can proceed.

Your assessment of the individual and the problem:

Your plan:

Your interventions:

Additional anticipatory planning:

Chapter 14 Psychological Therapies

ACTIVITY 1   Name _____

Case Study

Sally is a nursing student who verbalizes a concern that she is becoming overwhelmed by the stresses of being in school, working part-time to pay for her education, and living at home where her mother suffers from the debilitating effects of lupus erythematosus. She has made an appointment with an advanced practice psychiatric nurse to learn how to manage her stress more effectively.

List as many suggestions as you can for stress management techniques and lifestyle behaviors that will help Sally to cope with her situation in an adaptive way.

Chapter 14 Psychological Therapies

ACTIVITY 2   Name _____

....

Short Answer

1. Describe systematic or in vivo desensitization as it is used in the treatment of phobias and panic attacks.

2. What nursing responsibilities are associated with the implementation of treatment strategies in a behavioral model?

3. How are relaxation and biofeedback training used in a behavioral therapy model of treatment?

4. Explain classical and operant conditioning as they apply to behavioral therapy.

ACTIVITY 3   Name _____

Critical Thinking Exercise: Read the case study and answer the questions that follow.

Mrs. Anderson is a 48-year-old woman who has been brought to the mental health center by her husband because she has been refusing to eat for the past several days. She tells you that she must be punished because she is responsible for the sadness in the world as a result of her inability to be a good mother to her children. She says that they would have been better off if she had died years ago, and she thinks that her daughter's failure in school and marriage is her fault because she was too hard on her as a child. Mr. Anderson tells you that his wife is unable to sleep, seems really agitated, and sometimes talks as though she believes that her insides are "rotting away." He is very worried because she keeps saying that she deserves to die because she is so bad and that she will never feel any better than she does right now.

1. What negative thought processes and cognitive distortions contribute to the client's depression?

2. Describe how you would work with this client using a cognitive approach.

3. What evidence would demonstrate to you that your work with this client had been effective?

ACTIVITY 4   Name _____

Critical Thinking Exercise

Design an inpatient treatment unit for children with behavioral problems, using a behavior modification approach. Describe the unit's milieu, the activities available, the policies of the unit, the nursing responsibilities, and the reinforcement systems for appropriate behavior.

Chapter 15 Anxiety Disorders

ACTIVITY 1   Name _____

Match the level of anxiety from Column B to the symptom of anxiety in Column A. Items from Column B may be used more than once.

Column A   **Column B**

1. _____   Person is pale and experiencing hypotension.   a. mild

2. _____   Person feels threatened and startles easily.   b. moderate

3. _____   Person is aware of multiple environmental and   c. severe
            internal stimuli, with controlled thought
            processes.   d. panic

4. _____   Vital signs are slightly elevated.

5. _____   Person experiences excessive autonomic nervous
            system activity, including diaphoresis, urinary
            frequency and urgency, dry mouth, and dilated
            pupils.

6. _____   Pain and hearing sensations are minimal.

7. _____   Person feels energized—ready to face challenges
            and learn new skills.

8. _____   Problem-solving is difficult because of selective
            inattention.

9. _____   Person is relaxed and uses automatic or habitual
            behaviors

10. _____   Person feels helplessness and a total loss of
            control.

11. Explain the phenomenon of anxiety using the biological model and then compare that with the interpersonal model to describe the etiology of anxiety.

ACTIVITY 2   Name _____

....

Write in the blank the DSM-IV diagnosis that best fits the client described in each scenario. Use any of the following diagnoses.

panic disorder	generalized anxiety disorder
agoraphobia	obsessive-compulsive disorder
social phobia	dissociative amnesia
post-traumatic stress disorder	dissociative fugue
dissociative identity disorder	

Scenario #1   _____

Cynthia is worried because she has been experiencing numbness and tingling in her arms and hands, although her doctor tells her there is nothing physically wrong with her. When she has acute episodes of numbness and tingling, she also feels jittery, with hand tremors and weakness in her legs. She describes severe headaches, which feel like someone is tightening a metal band around her head. These episodes seem to come on for no apparent reason, and they last about 20 to 30 minutes before she feels all right again.

Scenario #2   _____

John finds himself counting cars in the parking lot before he can enter the building where he works. He feels that something really bad will happen if he doesn't count them. John knows that this is an irrational connection, but he can't get this thought out of his head and only feels better when he counts the cars.

Scenario #3   _____

Paul has been having nightmares every night for the past 6 months. He also notices that he startles easily, feels less like being around other people, and is drinking more alcohol than he used to. Paul describes himself as feeling numb and disconnected. He thinks this all began shortly after he responded to the site of a major airplane crash in his job as a paramedic.

Scenario #4   _____

The local news station has been featuring the picture of a woman, with a request that anyone who recognizes this woman should call the station to identify her. Apparently she has appeared in town and has no identification with her. She cannot remember who she is or where she came from. She seems to be upset about something.

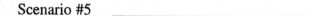

Sidney has taken a new job and finds himself extremely anxious about meeting new people and performing his work tasks with others watching. When he gets nervous around strangers at work, he notices chest pain, accompanied by palpitations and diaphoresis. He has begun thinking about calling in sick more frequently and worries that he will say or do something wrong.

Chapter 15 Anxiety Disorders

ACTIVITY 3   Name _____

Place an "X" in the blank beside those statements that are accurate and would be included in a teaching plan for a client with an anxiety disorder.

_____ 1. Differences in cultures affect manifestations of anxiety disorders.

_____ 2. Clients with anxiety disorders often experience other problems, too, such as depression, physical health problems, and substance abuse.

_____ 3. A phenomenon known as dyspareunia explains the neurotransmitter dysregulation involved in the anxiety disorders.

_____ 4. Well-adjusted individuals who have learned to manage stress effectively no longer experience anxiety because of their improved coping skills.

_____ 5. Medication is an effective part of the treatment plan and may involve drugs from either the antidepressant or the benzodiazepine categories.

_____ 6. Included in the treatment plan is the development of skill in various stress reduction techniques, such as progressive relaxation, deep breathing, and guided imagery.

_____ 7. Clients with anxiety disorders do not need to worry additionally about limiting their consumption of caffeine, alcohol, and nicotine, because these substances generally have a calming effect on an individual.

_____ 8. Benzodiazepines are the most effective medications available for the long-term relief of anxiety.

_____ 9. Two antidepressant medications that may be prescribed in the treatment of obsessive-compulsive disorder are clomipramine (Anafranil) and fluvoxamine (Luvox).

_____ 10. Clients who experience panic attacks can learn to identify their symptoms, situations that trigger those symptoms, and ways to restructure thought processes in order to control the body's physical response.

_____ 11. Seasonal changes in the time and duration of daylight and sunshine may trigger more frequent episodes of an anxiety disorder.

Develop a nursing care plan for the following client, using the blank form provided on the next page.

Susan is an 18-year-old college freshman being seen in the Student Counseling Center. She has been on edge since she left home 7 months ago to start school at a large urban university more than 4 hours away from her home in a small, rural town. She worries about everything she does at school and also worries about her mother and younger brother back home because she says her dad drinks too much and gets angry easily. Lately, Susan has been having difficulty concentrating on studying, and her grades are falling. She has trouble getting to sleep at night, and when she finally does sleep, it's rarely for more than 2 or 3 hours. She says her roommate is complaining that she is irritable all the time, but she thinks that is because she's always tired from lack of sleep. Susan says she's worried that she'll flunk out of school, but maybe that would be better so she could go home and take care of her family problems. She knows she would do much better in school if she stopped worrying so much, but she says she can't help herself.

Nursing Assessment Data

Nursing Diagnosis

Outcomes

    Short-term goals

    Long-term goals

  Interventions   **Rationale**

Chapter 16 Mood Disorders

ACTIVITY 1

Name _____

For the list of behaviors below, place an "X" in the second column if the behavior describes a person experiencing major depression without psychotic features. Place an "X" in the third column if the behavior describes a person experiencing bipolar disorder: mania.

Behavior	Major Depression	Bipolar Disorder: Mania
finds self sleeping all the time	X	
has spent several thousand dollars in past week		X
feels isolated and alone	X	
doesn't want to take time to eat		X
hears sounds inside head that seem to be voices		X
describes self as worthless	X	
is flirtatious and makes frequent sexual comments		X
talks in incoherent manner		X
feels tired all day	X	
doesn't recognize what to do with shoes		X
hasn't slept in several days	X	
reports difficulty concentrating on reading newspaper	X	
isn't interested in anything	X	X
feels really good	X	
startles easily		X
can't stop moving and talking		
has been less productive at work but keeps trying	X	
has lost weight recently and has no appetite	X	X
is disoriented to time and place		X
makes jokes frequently		
feels edgy and uneasy much of the time	X	

Behavior	Major Depression	Bipolar Disorder: Mania
jumps from topic to topic during conversation		X
doesn't want to make love with partner	X	
describes feelings of being hot, then cold		X
doesn't see any problems with behavior		X X
feels that others can read minds		
describes self as ugly, clumsy, and incompetent	X	
isn't worried about anything		X
is having increased difficulty with logic and reasoning		X X
is outgoing and social		X
seems highly suspicious of others		
has thought about ending life	X	
has been avoiding certain situations, such as going to the grocery store	X	
is easily distracted into another activity		X
can't remember names of family and co-workers		X
thinks and moves slowly	X	
has severe nausea, sometimes accompanied by diarrhea	X	X
thinks of self as very important and powerful		
describes a choking sensation in throat		
doesn't go out with friends anymore		
has been wearing bright colored clothing, with lots of makeup and jewelry		X

Chapter 16 Mood Disorders

ACTIVITY 2   Name _____

Short Answer

1. List at least five common physical health problems often associated with a mood disorder.

2. Describe the sleep disturbances associated with depression.

3. List at least five nursing diagnoses that are useful in directing nursing interventions for clients with mood disorders.

4. List at least five risk factors for suicide.

5. List at least five nursing interventions appropriate when working with an acutely suicidal client.

Chapter 16 Mood Disorders

ACTIVITY 3   Name _____

....

Critical Thinking Exercise: Read the case study and answer the questions that follow it.

Andrea is a 41-year-old single woman who is beginning a partial hospitalization program for help in learning to manage her feelings. She says that she has been sad most of her adult life but now feels hopeless and helpless because she has lost her mother. Andrea's mother died of pancreatic cancer approximately 9 months ago, and Andrea finds herself overwhelmed with sadness and feelings of guilt that she didn't do more to help her mother before her death. She is also worried that she will get very angry at her father (whom she describes as an alcoholic) and that she may hurt him.

Andrea lives at home with her father and brother. She has had to learn how to do the cooking and cleaning, as well as the other routine daily tasks that mother used to do for the family when she was alive. Andrea has not worked in the past 17 years, because she is in fragile physical health as a result of diabetes and hypothyroidism. She also admits being treated for bulimia years ago. Now when she gets really angry, she binges on junk food, which makes her blood sugar go up. Then she feels guilty, so she forces herself to vomit. She describes this pattern as occurring once per week or less but says she is more worried about her sadness.

Currently, Andrea sleeps only about 2 to 3 hours per night, and she forces herself to eat minimal amounts of food to keep her diabetes in control, even though she has no real appetite. She is apprehensive about joining the partial program because she doesn't like being around people and doesn't really enjoy any activities anymore. She says she would prefer to sit and watch.

1. List the symptoms for a mood disorder revealed in the case study.

2. What type of mood disorder is Andrea experiencing?

3. Identify key nursing interventions for Andrea.

4. What medication might you expect to be prescribed for Andrea, and what information would you need to teach her about it?

Chapter 16 Mood Disorders

ACTIVITY 4   Name _____

Critical Thinking Exercise: Read the case study and answer the questions that follow.

Alicia has been admitted to the short-stay psychiatric unit because her family found her running naked through the back yard, singing loudly. Alicia says she is feeling so good now that she doesn't need to sleep or eat. She just wants to have a good time and asks if the male nursing student can interview her so she can give him a few tips on success. She says she knows how to win friends and influence people because she has been to Carnegie Music Hall and has taken the Carnegie course on public speaking. She claims to have written a musical, which she is getting ready to take to Broadway, and that she is looking for people to star in it. Alicia is dressed in a bright red outfit with purple shoes and deep blue makeup. She has many bracelets and necklaces on, which she shakes dramatically when she wants to get someone's attention. When Alicia is asked to sit still so that the nurse can take her blood pressure, she gets angry and threatens to hit anyone who gets in her way. She constantly moves around the room, picking up objects to examine, then talking about something totally different than before. Alicia's family indicates that she has been like this for the past four days and that they are surprised she is not exhausted.

1. List the symptoms for a mood disorder revealed in the case study.

2. What type of mood disorder is Alicia experiencing?

3. Identify key nursing interventions for Alicia.

4. What medication might you expect to be prescribed for Alicia, and what information would you need to teach Alicia and her family about the medication?

Chapter 17 Substance Abuse

ACTIVITY 1   Name _____

Match the substance category from Column B to each substance in Column A.

Column A   **Column B**

1. _____ cocaine   a. CNS Depressant

2. _____ heroin   b. stimulant

3. _____ Valium   c. opioid

4. _____ LSD   d. hallucinogen

5. _____ alcohol   e. inhalant

6. _____ morphine

7. _____ nitrous oxide

8. _____ Benzedrine

9. _____ phenobarbital

10. _____ tetrahydrocannabinol

11. _____ methamphetamine

12. _____ Demerol

13. _____ mescaline

14. _____ caffeine

15. _____ Ritalin

16. _____ Dilaudid

17. _____ chloroform

18. _____ Seconal

19. _____ benzene

ACTIVITY 2   Name _____

....

Label each intervention with "P" for primary prevention and/or "T" for treatment of active problems. If you think that an intervention can be used in both of these stages, mark both.

_____ 1. Administer medication to control withdrawal symptoms.

_____ 2. Require client to attend problem-solving group.

_____ 3. Provide factual information regarding diagnosis and treatment.

_____ 4. Assist client to identify situations which lead to craving.

_____ 5. Assess for presence of medical complications.

_____ 6. Encourage family members to learn about substance abuse as a disease process.

_____ 7. Support measures to regulate the sale and distribution of alcohol to minors.

_____ 8. Provide quiet, calm, non-stimulating environment.

_____ 9. Assist client to obtain HIV testing if desired, and provide counseling when results are shared with client.

_____ 10. Instruct parents to develop and support school policies that prohibit alcohol and drug consumption at extracurricular activities.

_____ 11. Encourage client to become actively involved in therapeutic milieu on unit.

_____ 12. Assist client to identify substitute tension-reducing strategies.

_____ 13. Encourage responsible decision-making about lifestyle choices.

_____ 14. Assist client to identify use triggers.

_____ 15. Rehearse strategies for dealing with craving.

_____ 16. Identify high-risk individuals and institute measures to reduce the impact of risk factors.

_____ 17. Reinforce client's plan for aftercare, including regular attendance at 12-step meetings.

_____ 18. Work closely with other members of treatment team to minimize success of client's manipulative behavior.

_____ 19. Monitor client's response to withdrawal.

_____ 20. Teach junior high school students coping skills for dealing with peer pressure.

ACTIVITY 3   Name _____

....

Construct a nursing care plan to guide your work with the client described here. Use the blank form provided on the next page.

Mrs. Allen has been referred to the mental health clinic by her primary care physician because she has seemed depressed for the past several months. She has lost 20 pounds, even though her abdomen seems enlarged, and she reports that she is not interested in eating or any other kind of activity. She cries easily and makes no eye contact.

Mrs. Allen tells you that her sadness began approximately 4 years ago and has been getting worse these last 2 months. She hesitantly tells you that 4 years ago her little boy, age 2 at the time, wandered out of eyesight while she was talking on the phone. When she heard screeching automobile brakes, she rushed out of her house to find that he had been killed by a car driving down her street. Mrs. Allen has been overwhelmed by guilt since this event 4 years ago and has recently begun thinking about "just giving up on everything."

Mrs. Allen began drinking more frequently following the death of her son. She and her husband were fighting a lot, and she began having nightmares almost every night. She says the drinks soothed her nerves, helped her to sleep, and seemed to deaden her emotional pain to some extent. Now, she says, she drinks every day, often until she passes out. She wakes up wanting a drink and is terrified that she can't control her own behavior. Her husband has moved out, saying he can't stand watching what is happening, and Mrs. Allen says she now has no reason to go on living.

Nursing Assessment Data

Nursing Diagnosis

Outcomes

    Short-term goals

    Long-term goals

Interventions   **Rationale**

Chapter 17 Substance Abuse

ACTIVITY 4   Name _____

This activity is based on the video "Substance Abuse in Families, Children, and Adolescents"
from Mosby's Nursing Care of Clients with Substance Abuse Video Series.

1. List two ways the family with substance abuse attempts to survive.

2. In families with substance abuse, strong individuals often evolve to thwart the continuance of
   substance abuse.
   a. True
   b. False

3. State four ways codependence is damaging to the codependent.

4. The five role behaviors frequently assumed in families with substance abuse are chief enabler,

   _____, scapegoat, _____, and mascot.

5. List four problems experienced by children from families with a member who abuses substances.

6. When working with a child from a family with a member who abuses substances, the nurse
   should help the child develop coping skills as well as improve competence and

   _____.

7. Lack of parental supervision and poor parent-child relations place an adolescent at risk for substance abuse.
   a. True
   b. False

8. State the five strategies upon which prevention programs are based.

9. Not only do nurses identify substance abuse, but they help families face and deal with the problem, _____, and make referrals.

10. State two nursing diagnoses that might apply to an adolescent abusing substances.

Chapter 18 Cognitive and Organic Disorders

ACTIVITY 1   Name _____

Short Answer

1. Summarize the symptoms of delirium.

2. Summarize the symptoms of dementia.

3. List four possible causes of delirium.

4. List four possible causes of dementia.

5. Define the following terms:
   a. agnosia
   b. aphasia
   c. apraxia
   d. catastrophic reaction
   e. Sundowner's syndrome

Short Answer

1. List questions you would include in a comprehensive assessment of a client with possible dementia.

2. What instruments or assessment tools are available for the assessment of a client with possible dementia?

3. What diagnostic tests might provide helpful assessment data for a client with a cognitive impairment?

Chapter 18 Cognitive and Organic Disorders

ACTIVITY 3   Name _____

Discussion Questions: Within your clinical group or in the classroom in small groups, discuss your answers to the following questions. If this approach is not possible, write your own answers directly on this worksheet.

1. How would you design a residential facility for treatment of clients with dementia of the Alzheimer's type if you had no financial restrictions?

2. What resources exist in your geographical area for treatment of clients with dementia?

3. What communication techniques are effective when working with a client with dementia?

4. How can delirium related to alcohol withdrawal be prevented in a medical-surgical setting?

5. Describe nursing interventions appropriate for clients experiencing delirium.

Critical Thinking Exercise

David and Sherri have requested assistance in caring for his mother, Jane, who is 74 years old and is experiencing multiple cognitive deficits. Both David and Sherri work during the day. They check in on Jane each evening at her home where she lives with her husband Paul, a retired steelworker recovering from a heart attack and complications of diabetes. Sherri is tearful when she tells you that her mother-in-law sometimes doesn't recognize them and has wandered away from the house when frightened by something she doesn't understand. David is very quiet, but does admit that both he and his wife are exhausted and don't feel they have a life of their own anymore.

1. What help could you provide for David and Sherri?

2. What help may Jane and Paul need now or in the near future?

Chapter 19 Schizophrenia

ACTIVITY 1   Name _____

....

Complete the crossword puzzle, using the clues provided below.

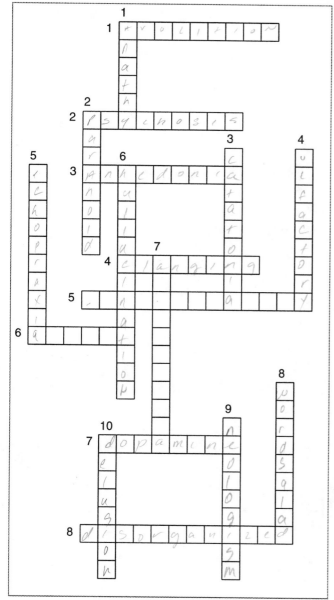

Across

1. no motivation to complete any task
2. having an impaired ability to recognize reality; unable to meet real world demands
3. loss of ability to enjoy things or experience pleasure
4. rhyming of words
5. getting off the subject when conversing
6. outward bodily expression of emotions
7. neurotransmitter affecting mood, affect, thoughts, behavior
8. type of schizophrenia characterized by severe disintegration, speech problems, odd behavior

Down

1. no interest, no feeling about anything
2. suspicious
3. intense motor disturbance characterizes a type of schizophrenia
4. kind of hallucination in which client smells something others do not
5. purposeless mimicking of other people's movements
6. subjective disorder of perception, involving one of the senses, in the absence of external stimuli
7. difficulty naming and describing emotions
8. the grouping of words together in a pattern which appears totally illogical and incoherent
9. the inventing of a word
10. false, fixed belief, resistant to reasoning, not based on verifiable facts

Chapter 19 Schizophrenia

Name _____

1. Give an example of the following symptoms of schizophrenia.

    a. auditory hallucination:

    b. persecutory delusion:

    c. looseness of association:

    d. incoherent use of language:

    e. difficulty sustaining attention:

    f. disorganized behavior:

    g. social dysfunction:

    h. grandiose delusion:

    i. thought broadcasting:

    j. poverty of speech:

2. Describe the neurobiological changes associated with schizophrenia.

ACTIVITY 3   Name _____

Critical Thinking Exercise: Read the case study and answer the questions that follow.

Sam is a 19-year-old who has been admitted to a psychiatric evaluation bed in a community hospital. You are assigned to provide primary care for him. When you first see him, you note that Sam has long, shaggy, and unwashed hair, that he is relatively thin, and that he makes no eye contact. He tells you, in a very soft voice, that Mary was supposed to care for him because he was nice to her, but she disappointed him by moving away. He is afraid that something is keeping them apart, and it may be because other people can read his thoughts. He says his thoughts are very loud, and they hurt him by bumping into the sides of his head. He asks you if you can hear his thoughts.

Sam has moved back into his parents' home, after living in a college dormitory for six months. He cannot remember if he is still enrolled in school, but he knows that he has not attended classes for several months, because "they won't help me make Mary understand." He believes that people at school want him to fail because they think he's not good enough for Mary, and he sees that some teachers wink at him to remind him that he is stupid. Sam says he has stopped caring about school and is not interested in getting a job because people there would keep him from being successful. He displays no emotion when telling you these things, and it appears to be hard for Sam to find the words to explain what he has been experiencing.

Sam seems easily distractible, constantly looking around the room, and moving restlessly in his seat. After only a few moments, he gets up and leaves the room.

1. Describe the symptoms that Sam displays.

2. Does Sam meet the DSM-IV criteria for schizophrenia?

3. What problems would you focus on if you were working with Sam in a therapeutic relationship?

Chapter 19 Schizophrenia

Name _____

Critical Thinking Exercise: Read the case study and answer the questions that follow.

Soon after she was married at the age of 20, Harriett was hospitalized for the first time. Her diagnosis was schizophrenia, and the hospital records noted that her behavior was silly, inappropriate, and childlike. Apparently, her thought processes and speech patterns had been hard to follow. Just prior to admission, her husband had found her in the kitchen putting vegetable peelings and cake batter on her head. She explained to him that there were spy cameras watching her all the time, and she was trying to fool them.

It has been 25 years since that first hospitalization, and Harriett has been hospitalized many times for similar problems. In between hospitalizations, she has lived at home, and her husband has looked after her. He has been leaving her a written schedule of what to do each hour of each day because he has found that she won't get out of bed if he doesn't structure her day for her.

Harriett's husband has brought her to the aftercare program because he is worried about her now. His job has changed, and he will be spending some time each month out of town. Because they have no children or other family and few friends, he thinks she needs someone to spend time with during the day. Harriett says she does not like to take medication, and she hopes that her attendance at this program will help her enough so that she does not need to take her pills. She wonders aloud whether the building is "haunted" and smiles inappropriately.

1. Describe Harriett's symptoms.

2. What are the problems faced by many clients, like Harriett, with severe and persistent mental disorders?

3. How can you help Harriett to get involved in the aftercare program? What services or activities might be of most interest and benefit to Harriett?

4. How would you ensure continuity of care for Harriett and other clients like her?

Chapter 20 Somatoform Disorders

ACTIVITY 1   Name _____

....

Match the diagnosis from the "Somatoform Disorders" category of DSM-IV in Column A with the description of the disorder in Column B.

Column A   **Column B**

_____ 1. somatization disorder   a. preoccupation with fears of having a serious disease based on misinterpretation of bodily symptoms

_____ 2. hypochondriasis

_____ 3. body dysmorphic disorder   b. pain in more than one anatomical site, causing significant distress and impaired functioning

_____ 4. conversion disorder
                                        c. history of many physical complaints, including at least four pain symptoms, two gastrointestinal symptoms, one sexual symptom, and one neurological symptom
_____ 5. pain disorder

                                        d. preoccupation with a real or imagined defect in appearance

                                        e. one or more deficits affecting voluntary motor or sensory functioning, associated with a psychological stressor

6. List 10 physical conditions affected by psychological factors, often called psychophysiological illnesses.

Chapter 20 Somatoform Disorders

ACTIVITY 2   Name _____

Discussion Questions: Within your clinical group or in the classroom in small groups, discuss your answers to the following questions. If this approach is not possible, write your own answers directly on this worksheet.

1. Clients with somatoform disorders and other psychophysiological diseases often experience excessive amounts of stress. Explain the connection between stress and the development of physical symptoms.

2. How would you assess a client who is reporting chronic pain?

3. Describe some strategies clients can use to improve sleep patterns.

4. Identify psychological responses to chronic health problems that may require some nursing interventions to help the client cope more effectively.

5. What medications may be ordered to help a client who is experiencing anxiety symptoms? What should the client and family be taught about these medications?

6. List some teaching points to include to help clients and families adjust psychologically to an acute illness.

Chapter 20 Somatoform Disorders

ACTIVITY 3   Name _____

Place an "X" in the blank beside each nursing intervention that would be a part of a care plan to help increase a client's ability to cope with stress and anxiety.

_____ 1. Orient the client to reality frequently.

_____ 2. Take resting pulse, blood pressure, and respirations.

_____ 3. Assess current level of anxiety.

_____ 4. Stay with person and do not make any demands on him or her.

_____ 5. Establish a trusting relationship.

_____ 6. Maintain adequate nutrition and hydration.

_____ 7. Provide support and encouragement to promote success.

_____ 8. Evaluate all abnormal lab findings.

_____ 9. Convey a sense of empathy and understanding.

_____ 10. Encourage expression of feelings.

_____ 11. Keep client's door closed at all times.

_____ 12. Ask questions, but do not wait for client's answer.

_____ 13. Give detailed directions so that client is clear about what to do.

_____ 14. Avoid physical contact with client.

_____ 15. Assess client's current coping skills.

_____ 16. Encourage client to evaluate own behavior.

_____ 17. Initiate referrals as needed.

_____ 18. Encourage socialization.

_____ 19. Acknowledge physical symptoms without undue emphasis.

_____ 20. Teach new coping skills, like relaxation and assertiveness.

_____ 21. Set limits on inappropriate behavior.

_____ 22. Distract client from grandiose thinking.

_____ 23. Help client express feelings about conflicts.

_____ 24. Provide information about healthy lifestyle.

_____ 25. Reduce gains from "sick role."

Chapter 20 Somatoform Disorders

ACTIVITY 4   Name _____

Critical Thinking Exercise: Read the case study and answer the questions that follow.

Mrs. S is a 38-year-old, married female, who is currently in a wheelchair because she claims she cannot walk. She has also experienced weakness in her arms, clenched fists without being able to extend her fingers, and frequent episodes of dropping objects. Her primary care physician referred her to a neurologist for a complete diagnostic workup, and all of her tests were within normal limits. She has been sent to the psychiatric medicine clinic for a psychiatric assessment, and during the interview, she tells you that she has been in this wheelchair since she was assaulted by a student in her workplace. Apparently, she was badly beaten and required surgery to repair a broken jaw. Mrs. S says this is nothing new, because she has been beaten by both parents all her life. She says she was so angry at the student that she thought she could kill him, and that awareness has her terribly frightened.

1. What psychiatric diagnosis might Mrs. S receive? Why?

2. What additional data would you like to collect?

3. List three nursing diagnoses that reflect the priorities you see in working with Mrs. S.

4. What nursing interventions would be a part of your care plan?

5. Do you anticipate any problems for Mrs. S's family? How would you help family members to understand Mrs. S's illness?

Chapter 21 Personality Disorders

ACTIVITY 1   Name _____

....

Identify the correct DSM-IV cluster for each of the personality disorders listed below.

Personality Disorder   **Cluster**

_____ 1. obsessive-compulsive   a. eccentric

_____ 2. schizoid   b. erratic

_____ 3. histrionic   c. fearful

_____ 4. borderline

_____ 5. paranoid

_____ 6. dependent

_____ 7. narcissistic

_____ 8. schizotypal

_____ 9. antisocial

_____ 10. avoidant

Column A contains descriptions of each of the 10 diagnoses in the "Personality Disorders" (PD) category of DSM-IV. Match the diagnosis in Column B with the corresponding personality description in Column A.

Column A	Column B
_____ 11. superstitious, believes in magic, ideas of reference	a. paranoid PD
	b. borderline PD
_____ 12. submissive, clinging, unable to make decisions by self	c. dependent PD
_____ 13. intense relationships, self-mutilation, impulsiveness	d. narcissistic PD
	e. schizoid PD
_____ 14. preoccupied with perfection, conscious of rules, self-critical, controlling	f. avoidant PD
_____ 15. grandiose view of self, lacks empathy for others	g. obsessive-compulsive PD
	h. histrionic PD
_____ 16. doesn't want to socialize, prefers to be alone, detached	i. antisocial PD
_____ 17. irresponsible, displays lack of guilt, good at manipulation	j. schizotypal PD
_____ 18. suspicious, jealous, short-tempered, unwilling to problem-solve	
_____ 19. fearful of criticism and rejection, negative self-esteem, few social interactions	
_____ 20. attention-seeking, self-centered, seductive, dramatic	

Chapter 21 Personality Disorders

ACTIVITY 2   Name _____

....

Discussion Questions: Within your clinical group or in the classroom, discuss your answers to the following questions. If this approach is not possible, write your own answers directly on this worksheet.

1. Describe how traits associated with obsessive-compulsive personality disorder can help some people perform their jobs better, whereas for others the same traits or exaggerated versions of the traits become a problem causing significant distress.

2. Define manipulation and give some examples of manipulative behavior clients might display. Are there some situations in which—or some clients by which—you might be more easily manipulated? What feelings do manipulative clients evoke in you, and how can you manage those feelings?

3. Describe the process of setting limits. What kinds of clients need firm limits and structure? How can a staff deal with clients who repeatedly test the limits? What are some problems that may occur in a unit or program that is unable to successfully set limits?

Chapter 21 Personality Disorders

ACTIVITY 3   Name _____

For each situation, read the client data and the nursing diagnosis, then suggest three nursing interventions that would be essential when working with this client.

Situation #1

Data: The client is 24 year old and single. She has been living with her grandmother since age 13 when her mother threw her out. She came to the psychiatric unit after entering the hospital via the ER with a gun-shot to abdomen. She claims the gunshot was not a suicide attempt, but rather an effort to punish her boyfriend for arriving late to give her a ride to work. The client demands a primary nurse who will be available at all times to help her solve her family problems.

Nursing Diagnosis: High risk for violence: self-directed

Nursing Interventions:

1.

2.

3.

Situation #2

Data: The client is a 42-year-old, single female, living in family home with her alcoholic father and unemployed brother. She says she is severely depressed since her mother died several months ago from pancreatic cancer. She has no friends and prefers to be alone. She says she has always been that way and that she can remember playing with dolls and making up fantasies so she didn't have to go out of the house. The client has been unable to complete ADL's. She says her mother did everything for the family, and she doesn't know how to cook or clean. The client knows she needs help to over come her depressive symptoms, but she can't bring herself to attend a day treatment center, because there are too many people there. She says she wouldn't feel safe or comfortable.

Nursing Diagnosis: Impaired social interaction

Nursing Interventions:

1.

2.

3.

Situation #3

Data: The client is a 31-year-old male, court-ordered for treatment. He entered treatment via the ER, where he was treated for broken ribs and multiple cuts, sustained during a bar fight. The client has had three brief marriages, and he does not provide any financial support to any of his ex-wives. He says they knew what they were getting into when they married him. The client has been observed alternating very charming behavior with angry outbursts. He demands to be able to smoke on the unit, even though it is a nonsmoking facility—he says "rules are made to be broken." The client has a history of multiple admissions for treatment of alcohol abuse but refuses to quit drinking—he says he likes the way he lives.

Nursing Diagnosis: Ineffective individual coping

Nursing Interventions:

1.

2.

3.

Chapter 21 Personality Disorders

ACTIVITY 4   Name _____

Critical Thinking Questions

1. One of your clients is a 20-year-old female, who has been admitted with the following diagnoses:
   Axis I: Major depression (single episode), moderate anorexia nervosa
   Axis II: Borderline personality disorder

   What will be your priorities for care while this client is an inpatient?

2. The evening staff is upset because they have heard from one of the unit's clients that the daylight staff is complaining about them. The client says that the evening staff is being blamed for the unit looking messy and the paperwork not being completed. The nurses who work evenings are angry because they feel that it is the daylight staff who don't complete their paperwork. You notice that the same client, Mr. Allen, is talking to the staff on both shifts, telling stories about the other staff and feeding their anger. This client has also been observed spending large amounts of time alone in his room, even when he is supposed to be in group, but it seems as though the staff is too busy fighting with each other to notice Mr. Allen's behavior. If the unit had access to a clinical nurse specialist, what interventions might be made to improve this situation?

3. You are making home visits in a community health nursing course. One of your clients is a 48-year-old woman who has been diagnosed as having dependent personality disorder. Her husband is an alcoholic who has not yet sought treatment, and her daughter has been "experimenting with drugs in order to feel better." The youngest child has a severe physical handicap that has required the family to make many adaptations. Your client says she would do anything to help her family.

   What are your priorities in working with this client and the whole family system?

ACTIVITY 1   Name _____

Describe the factors that influence the development of eating disorders, using each of the categories listed below.

1. Biological

2. Genetic

3. Intrapersonal/Interpersonal

4. Family

5. Sociocultural

Chapter 22 Eating Disorders

ACTIVITY 2   Name _____

Label each piece of data below with "A" if it describes someone with anorexia and "B" if it describes someone with bulimia. Both "A" and "B" may be used if the data would be found in persons with either disorder.

1. _____self-starvation, refusal to eat

2. _____hypokalemia

3. _____parotid gland enlargement

4. _____constant striving for the "perfect" body

5. _____denial of seriousness of current low weight

6. _____weight at least 15% below ideal weight

7. _____cardiac arrhythmia/dysrhythmia

8. _____dental enamel erosion

9. _____constipation

10. _____cachexia

11. _____amenorrhea

12. _____preoccupation with food

13. _____body image disturbance

14. _____seeing fat when actually emaciated

15. _____dehydration

16. _____cardiomyopathy

17. _____slow pulse

18. _____decreased body temperature

19. _____excessive use of laxatives, diuretics, enemas

20. _____recurrent binge eating of large amounts of food

21. _____Mallory-Weiss tears in esophagus

Chapter 22 Eating Disorders

ACTIVITY 3   Name _____

Critical Thinking Exercise: Read the case study and answer the questions that follow.

Abby is a 19-year-old beauty school student who has been brought to the ER by her roommate, because apparently Abby collapsed, unconscious, in the bathroom. The roommate, Ellen, says she thinks this all happened because Abby is starving herself. Ellen says she never sees Abby eat, and she has noticed that all of Abby's clothes just hang loosely on her. Ellen describes Abby as very defensive about her appearance, and very secretive in her behavior. Ellen doesn't know much else about Abby or her family, except that it seems as though Abby feels she has to look and be perfect in order to satisfy her parents.

1. Summarize what you know about Abby.

2. What additional data would you collect in order to complete a comprehensive nursing assessment on Abby?

3. What nursing diagnoses are you likely to identify?

4. Explain how you would intervene with Abby.

Chapter 22 Eating Disorders

Name _____

Critical Thinking Exercise

You have been asked to provide a program on eating disorders for the PTA at the local elementary school. If you wanted to emphasize prevention as well as treatment, what content would you include in your presentation?

Chapter 23 Sexual Disorders

ACTIVITY 1   Name _____

Unscramble the words or phrases associated with sexual responses and dysfunctions, using the clues provided.

1. P A S U I Y D R A N E
    _____   genital pain associated with sexual intercourse

2. M D S S I A
    _____   sexual arousal achieved by inflicting pain on someone else

3. R Y I O V U M E S
    _____   arousal achieved by observing an unsuspecting person naked, in the act of disrobing, or engaging in sexual activity

4. A P H L I I A A R P S
    _____   group of behaviors commonly known as sexual deviations

5. H E A I P O P I L D
    _____   fondling or other sexual activity with a child under age 13

6. S G A S U N I V M I
    _____   involuntary contractions of perineal muscles with penetration

7. B I E M S O T X I I H N I
    _____   exposure of one's genitals to an unsuspecting person, followed by sexual arousal

8. V T A S T R E S T E I N
    _____   person who is sexually aroused by cross-dressing

9. C A O M M S S I H
    _____   sexual arousal achieved by being receiver of pain, humiliation

10. T M P R A U E R E
    T N A L C E O A I U J   onset of orgasm and release of semen with minimal sexual stimulation
    _____

11. Distinguish between sexual dysfunction and sexual deviation.

Chapter 23 Sexual Disorders

ACTIVITY 2

Name _____

Discussion Questions: Within your clinical group or in the classroom, discuss your answers to the following questions. If this approach is not possible, write your own answers directly on this worksheet.

1. You have been asked to do a presentation on healthy sexual behaviors and/or activities for a health class of high school juniors. What content would you include?

2. What questions would you include in an assessment of sexuality and sexual behaviors?

3. Some of your clients are at risk for developing HIV. What information about sexual activity will you provide for them?

4. How can you create a climate within a nurse-client relationship that helps the client feel comfortable asking you about sexual issues?

Chapter 23 Sexual Disorders

ACTIVITY 3   Name _____

Critical Thinking Activity: Consider the following data and nursing diagnoses, then write three nursing interventions for each situation.

Situation #1

    Data: The husband is 35; the wife is 34. Both are in good physical health. The wife is being treated for depression and is taking an antidepressant. They describe their sexual relationship as good until first child was born. He wants physical intimacy more frequently. She says she is not interested in sexual activity but would like more tenderness. The frequency of their sexual activity has become approximately 1 times per month.

    Nursing Diagnosis: Sexual dysfunction

    Nursing Interventions:

1.

2.

3.

Situation #2

    Data: The client is a 26-year-old female, diagnosed with borderline personality disorder. She reports a history of sexual abuse and physical abuse by several male members of her family while growing up. She currently describes sexual arousal as dependent on being handled aggressively, burned, cut, or urinated on by her partner.

    Nursing Diagnosis: Disturbance in self-concept: self-esteem

    Nursing Interventions:

1.

2.

3.

Situation #3

Data: The client has come to the mental health center for evaluation of depression. She states that she feels guilty and is afraid she will go to hell. She expresses anger at God for allowing her to get herself into this "bad" situation. She reluctantly admits to having sexual activity with another female, which she enjoyed, and also masturbating in between times she sees this other woman.

Nursing Diagnosis: Spiritual distress

Nursing Interventions:

1.

2.

3.

Chapter 24 Children and Adolescents

ACTIVITY 1   Name _____

1. List at least five risk factors that contribute to the development of childhood psychiatric disorders.

2. Describe resiliency, and list factors that enhance resiliency in children and adolescents.

3. Match the description of the disorder generally occurring in childhood with the corresponding diagnosis from DSM-IV.

_____ mental retardation

_____ motor skills disorder

_____ elimination disorder

_____ attention deficit disorder

_____ tic disorders

_____ separation anxiety

a. excessive difficulty leaving home or people to whom the child is attached

b. involuntary, sudden, recurrent, stereotyped movement or vocalization

c. significantly subaverage intellectual functioning

d. coordination substantially below expectation for age

e. repeated passage of feces in inappropriate places after age 4

f. maladaptive behaviors related to inattention

Chapter 24 Children and Adolescents

ACTIVITY 2   Name _____

1. List three medications used to treat psychiatric disorders in children, and describe what they are used for.

2. Describe treatment methods that are uniquely used to work therapeutically with children.

3. List nursing interventions for each of the following nursing diagnoses that may be made after analyzing data about a child with some type of psychiatric disorder.

   a. Altered family processes

   b. Altered growth and development

   c. Anxiety

   d. Body image disturbance

   e. Chronic low self-esteem

   f. Impaired social interaction

   g. Risk for violence

Chapter 24 Children and Adolescents

ACTIVITY 3   Name _____

....

Discussion Questions: Within your clinical group or in the classroom, discuss your answers to the following questions. If this approach is not possible, write your own answers directly on this worksheet.

1. Describe the profile of the high-risk adolescent.

2. Describe the criteria for making a diagnosis of conduct disorder.

3. What are some clues that might indicate that an adolescent is suicidal?

4. Discuss the issue of teen-age violence. What are some factors that contribute to it? How would you intervene to prevent violence by adolescents?

5. Identify several sexuality-related problems that may occur during adolescence, causing difficulty in adjustment.

ACTIVITY 4   Name _____

Critical Thinking Exercise: Read the case study and answer the questions that follow.

Paula is a 14-year-old female who has been admitted to the inpatient adolescent unit with the following symptoms: persistent sadness, suicidal thoughts accompanied by the beginning of a suicide plan, refusal to eat, difficulty falling asleep and staying asleep, feelings of hopelessness, lack of energy, slowed body movements and thought processes, difficulty concentrating, lack of enjoyment of any activities. Paula has been accompanied by her aunt, who is apparently raising Paula since her parents were arrested for drug distribution. Paula's aunt reluctantly divulges that Paula has been severely abused, both physically and sexually, and has been neglected by her parents from the time she was born. She has been having trouble in school and does not seem to have any friends.

1. From an analysis of this data about Paula, what problems can you identify?

2. What additional data will you collect?

3. What will be your initial priority in providing care for Paula?

4. List five key nursing interventions for Paula.

5. What kinds of interventions may be necessary after inpatient treatment is completed?

Chapter 25 The Elderly

ACTIVITY 1   Name _____

Read each statement about the elderly and indicate a "T" for True and an "F" for False.

_____ 1. The group of people in this country who are age 85 or older are in the fastest growing population group.

_____ 2. Elderly persons have worse dietary habits and consume more tobacco products and alcohol than do younger people.

_____ 3. Depression is the most common mental disorder in the elderly, but it is often overlooked, misdiagnosed, and inadequately treated.

_____ 4. Many medications that the elderly person may be taking can contribute to depression.

_____ 5. Elderly persons are not physically able to maintain sexual activity and are generally not interested anyway.

_____ 6. Elderly persons with decreased cognitive abilities may experience feelings of powerlessness, anger, and low self-esteem.

_____ 7. Cognitive processes do not decline simply because of the aging process.

_____ 8. Depression in the elderly is inevitable because they experience so many losses.

_____ 9. Loneliness and isolation are not problems for the elderly as they age if they have been reasonably active during their adult work years.

_____ 10. All elderly persons with mental disorders are in nursing homes because they require institutional care.

Chapter 25 The Elderly

ACTIVITY 2   Name _____

Complete the sentences below, using the following words and phrases.

reality orientation   pet therapy
reminiscence therapy   ageism
altered pharmacokinetics   milieu management
geropsychiatric nursing   short-term memory
Short Portable Mental Status Questionnaire   Geriatric Depression Scale

1. _____ results when the aging process produces numerous bodily changes that alter the absorption, distribution, metabolism, and excretion of drugs.

2. A specific type of therapy, in which the nurse uses bulletin boards with information about the day, date, next meal, next holiday, and weather that is helpful in keeping the elderly person in touch with what is currently happening, is known as _____.

3. _____ is the dislike of and discrimination against the elderly by some caregivers, creating a barrier to effective treatment.

4. An effective tool for assessing the presence of profound sadness in an elderly person is the _____.

5. The nurse who is doing _____ would ask elderly clients to share with a group of their peers their memories of events from the past, such as vacations, family experiences, and special occasions.

6. If the nurse is assessing an elderly person's cognitive abilities, he or she might use the _____.

7. The ability to remember the recent past is known as _____.

8. A specialty in which the nurse has in-depth knowledge about the elderly and also about mental disorders is known as _____.

9. The careful design of the environment to support meaningful interaction and maintenance of functional ability is known as _____.

10. When the nurse wants to break through an elderly person's depression and apathy, she may try _____ by bringing in an animal for the client to hold and talk to.

Chapter 25 The Elderly

ACTIVITY 3   Name _____

Discussion Questions: Within your clinical group or in the classroom, discuss your answers to the following questions. If this approach is not possible, write your own answers directly on this worksheet.

1. Describe the functional assessment of an elderly person. What data will you collect, and how will you accomplish this phase of the nursing process?

2. Describe physical and psychological changes that are a normal part of the aging process.

3. How does a nurse's attitude toward aging and the elderly person affect the care provided?

4. Identify key components of a mental status examination of an elderly person, and describe one assessment tool.

ACTIVITY 4   Name _____

....

Critical Thinking Exercise: Read the case study and answer the questions that follow.

Mrs. E. is a 77-year-old widow, who lives in a retirement apartment complex. Her husband died of a heart attack 10 years ago, and she has been in this apartment since then. Mrs. E. had a heart attack 8 years ago, and she has recovered well. Recently, she developed severe abdominal pain, radiating around to her back. This pain has awakened her several times during the night, and she is quite frightened. She has called the visiting nurse to come see her, and today she tells the nurse that she thinks she may be having a heart attack like she had before. She says that she is unable to sleep at night, feels jittery all the time, and wants to call her children, who live several hours from her, to tell them that she is sorry for anything she may have done wrong while they were growing up. She says she wants to make amends before dying.

1. What do you currently know about Mrs. E?

2. What additional data do you need to collect?

3. What problems can you identify, based on the data you have?

4. List key nursing interventions to support Mrs. E.

Chapter 26 Vulnerable Populations

ACTIVITY 1   Name _____

Critical Thinking Exercise: Read the case study and answer the questions that follow.

Anna is a 78-year-old woman who has been brought to the emergency room with chest pain and shortness of breath. She is accompanied by her daughter and son-in-law. Her daughter is reluctant to leave her mother's side, but her son-in-law leaves quickly and says he'll be back later. Anna has been on medication for treatment of angina, and with some prompt intervention in the ER, she is stabilized. The nurse asks the daughter to wait in the visitor's lounge while she finishes the paperwork for Anna's discharge. When Anna is alone, the nurse completes a psychosocial assessment. Anna has been living with her daughter and son-in-law for about a year, since her husband died. She has difficulty making eye contact, seems very sad, and indicates that she feels isolated and lonely. With some gentle questioning, Anna admits that she has been uncomfortable in her daughter's house, because she thinks that she is not wanted there. She says they don't take her anywhere, so she spends most of her time in her bedroom. On several occasions, when she asked for something she needed, they yelled at her, and her son-in-law hit her hard, leaving bruises. She says they don't mean to treat her badly but they are "under a lot of stress and they often drink more than they should." Anna says she is most worried that something will happen to her because of her heart problems and that they won't do anything about it.

1. What nursing diagnoses might you consider based on what you know about Anna and her situation?

2. What kinds of questions might the nurse have asked to elicit the data needed about Anna's living situation?

3. Describe a comprehensive assessment of an elderly person if abuse is suspected.

4. What interventions would you make in this situation?

Chapter 26 Vulnerable Populations

ACTIVITY 2

Name _____

....

Critical Thinking Exercise: Read the case study and answer the questions that follow.

Sue is a 42-year-old woman who has presented in a psychiatric outpatient clinic for an evaluation of depression. She indicates the following symptoms: sleep and appetite disturbances, constipation, chronic back and neck pains, migraine headaches, occasional heart palpitations, dizziness, and persistent sadness. She says she is not sure why she came, because she is convinced that things can never be any better. She has been taking antianxiety medication prescribed by her family doctor, but she says it hasn't helped. She tells you that she used to work as a medical laboratory researcher, but she quit two months ago to be a full-time mother to her 2- and 5-year-old boys. She says they are a handful, because they are both fairly hyperactive. She says her husband, a college professor, thinks that she should be more strict with the boys and not let them take advantage of her. Sue indicates that her husband works very long hours on his research and is not home to help her. She says when he does come home, he gets a beer and watches TV all evening. She says she doesn't want him to know that she has come to the clinic, because he wouldn't approve. You notice that Sue is soft-spoken, hesitant, and dressed in long-sleeved clothing even though it is warm today.

1. How would you describe the problems that Sue may be having?

2. If you suspected that Sue might be a victim of domestic violence, how would you assess her further? What clues would you look for?

3. What characteristics are associated with a batterer or perpetrator of violence?

4. Identify outcomes for Sue as a result of nursing interventions.

5. List five interventions you would make with a client who is experiencing domestic violence.

Critical Thinking Exercise: Read the case study and answer the questions that follow.

Matt is a 26-year-old computer analyst who has been referred for a psychiatric assessment because his primary care physician has noticed a persistent sad mood while treating Matt's severe headaches for the past several months. Matt reveals sufficient symptoms to meet the criteria for a diagnosis of major depression, recurrent episode, severe. He indicates that he was treated for depression as an early teenager, then again as a freshman in college, and he is extremely distressed that the depression is back now. He is worried because his job is being eliminated in six months, and he is also upset because he has just broken off a relationship with a homosexual partner of 6 years to start a new relationship with another man. Matt says he feels guilty all the time and is very sad because his parents don't accept his sexual preferences. But, he says, these stressors don't bother him as much as the nightmares he has several nights a week that wake him up screaming. With some prompting, he reveals that the nightmares are a reenactment of childhood sexual abuse that he experienced for 4 years, from 5th grade to 9th grade, perpetrated by his boy scout leader. Matt says he has been drinking more than he wants to lately, because he finds that getting drunk is the only way he can sleep and forget about all of his difficulties.

1. Describe childhood sexual abuse. What forms can it take, and how many people does it affect?

2. What adult problems are noted in people who have experienced childhood sexual abuse?

3. Identify three problems that Matt is experiencing.

4. Suggest three interventions that would benefit Matt.

Chapter 26 Vulnerable Populations

ACTIVITY 4   Name _____

....

Critical Thinking Exercise: Read the case study and answer the questions that follow.

Raymond is a 46-year-old man with a history of complex partial seizures that have required treatment for more than 30 years. Ray lives with his mother but indicates that he does not get along with her at all. He would like to live alone, but he feels unable to because of his seizure disorder. He has been treated before for depression and says that he was court-committed at that time. He is not sure how that happened; all that he can remember is that he called a suicide hotline, and the next thing he knew, the police were taking him to the hospital. He has been referred for assessment and treatment because his neurologist has noted a recurrence of symptoms associated with depression. Ray does agree that he is feeling guilty that he hates his mother and angry that he has to stay with her. He says he also feels sad, self-conscious, and chronically tired. Ray also admits to anhedonia, anergia, lack of appetite, and difficulty falling asleep.

1. What risk factors are associated with an increased risk for suicide?

2. How would you assess Ray for suicide ideation or plan?

3. What is the priority when working with a client with moderate or high suicide risk?

4. List three nursing interventions you would make with Ray.